Table of Contents

Understanding the Relationship Between Joint Pain and Weakness: 7 Conditions and Treatment Strategies

Understanding Joint Pain and Weakness: Causes, Symptoms, and Treatment

1. Introduction to Joint Pain and Weakness

Activities such as arthritis management or balance and gait training can be included in an exercise routine to help increase joint health. Exercises focusing on re-education of working muscles around a joint can help decrease stiffness, increase strength, and improve flexibility. Chiropractic adjustments, cold laser therapy, or low-dose medications may also be used to decrease your joint pain. Orthotics or joint braces could be used with input from a qualified healthcare provider to help stabilize the joint. Injections or radiofrequency ablation (burning procedure) may be helpful for some patients. Keeping a food journal and being mindful of how dietary habits affect your energy and overall feeling is important as well. Nutritional counseling can be helpful to meet your individual needs. Always start a new exercise or nutrition program under the guidance of a professional.

This essay will discuss the causes, symptoms, and treatment options for joint pain and weakness, which may contribute to an overall sense of unwellness and decreased mobility. Joint health is important in maintaining mobility across the lifespan, and it is important to understand changes in joint health as they relate to overall health and functioning. This essay contains general information and may be helpful to anyone, not just those who have pain or weakness in their joints. Please consult with a professional for individualized recommendations.

2. Anatomy of Joints

Joints exist in specific parts of the human body. Some of them are common to both the upper and lower extremities. The shoulder, elbow, wrist, hip, knee, and ankle all contain the same types of joints. They possess the basic elements of a joint: articular cartilage, synovial fluid, synovial membrane, hyaline cartilage or fibrocartilage, and ligaments. The articular cartilage is found on the surfaces of the bones. It acts as a cushion between the bones and a lubricant. It provides the smooth surface needed for movement, and it helps to distribute body weight and reduce friction. The ligaments are like the duct tape for the bones that help to hold everything in place. They are strong and flexible. Injuries that damage or tear the soft tissue structures (ligaments) that connect and support the joint and surrounding musculature are called "sprains." In most cases, strains are caused by accidents, violence, or sports. Roughly five to ten per five thousand people in the United States have a sprain or strain at any given time, according to the CDC.

Joints are anatomical structures that facilitate movement and support and connect different bones and tissues in the human body. They make every possible movement and some other functions possible for a person. Broadly, there are three major types of joints: synovial, cartilaginous, and fibrous. Synovial joints consist of a prominent joint capsule that contains synovial fluid. This fluid helps to reduce friction and minimize wear and tear during movement. A cartilaginous joint is a connection between two bones made of cartilage. They allow for more movement between the bones and ligaments that hold them in place. The bones do not actually touch; the contractions of the surrounding musculature keep them stable. Fibrous joints are connected together by strong connective tissue, namely ligaments, which makes them extremely stable. They don't have nerves inside the cartilage and form synovial joints.

2.1. Types of Joints

- Hinge joints (elbow, knee) - Pivot joints (neck, forearm) - Saddle joints (thumb) - Ball-and-socket joints (shoulder, hip) - Ellipsoidal joints (wrist)

- Fibrous (immobile) - Cartilaginous (slightly movable) - Synovial (freely movable) which include subtypes:

Different types of joints include the following:

Joints can be classified according to their structure or function. Based on structure, there are three major categories of joints: fibrous (syndesmoses), cartilaginous (synchondroses), and synovial. These three categories can be divided into even more specialized types based on the type of tissue and eventual function. Most joints are mobile, allowing movement at the point where bones meet. In general, the greater the range of motion, the fewer the number of ligaments a joint has.

A joint is a point at which two bones meet. It allows for movement of the body or a part of the body. Several different types of joints allow for different degrees and types of movement.

2.2. Function of Joints

Joints can be of many types and subtypes and each is specific to providing hyper specific motions. For example, the hinge joint at the elbow and knee are uniaxial, meaning they perform rotation in only one plane and one axis, the flexion/extension range of motion i.e in the sagittal plane. Similarly, the saddle joint at the carpometacarpal joints of the thumb allows all movements, which also includes opposing the extremities or the range of motions of other joints. The pivot joint at the atlas-axis of the neck enables one bone to rotate around the long axis of the other. At the glenohumeral joint at the shoulder, the ball-and-socket joint enables all movements, but because of the deep articulating cavity and strong ligaments that hold the joint, it is also the most mobile yet least stable joint in the body. In the same way, the hip joint and the ankle joint differ in biomechanics, just as the movements they provide also differ. Having observed the functioning of ball-and-socket, hinge, pivot and saddle joints of the skeletal system, one tends to think of the fascinating biomechanics of the diverse movements they enable.

Joints play a cardinal and indispensable role in the musculoskeletal system. Their presence allows for the articulation of bones with one another, helping the skeletal structure to effect movements. In humans, different types of joints enable a range of movements right from simple angular movements to the more complex specialized synovial movements and not to forget the pivotal movements of the bony supports of the axial body and appendicular skeleton. Joints possess the ability to bear the body weight and perform whatever movement they are capable of performing.

3. Causes of Joint Pain and Weakness

Probably the most common cause of joint pain and weakness, inflammation can last for a short duration, resolve over time, and not be so severe or severe for chronic types that can have an enormous impact on everyday life. Infectious factors include when infections, septic arthritis, or viral infections travel from other areas of the body and stop in the joints. Osteoarthritis causes the wearing away and subsequent roughening of the cartilage that covers the surface of the joints. It is the most common type of arthritis and women again are at a higher risk for developing this condition.

Joint pain and weakness can result from a variety of different factors, many of which are due to injuries or chronic conditions. These same factors that can commonly cause pain in the joints also apply to weakness. One of the most common causes of pain in the affected area is inflammation. This is your body's natural protective response that occurs when tissues are injured, such as during a sprained elbow, a broken bone, or when you have a sports-related injury that affects this area. However, inflammation can also have its origins from a longer-lasting condition, such as arthritis, which is the leading cause of joint pain and weakness. Pain in this area and weakness in the affected joints can also be caused by the cartilage that covers the articular surfaces becoming worn away over time, which is the case for people who have osteoarthritis deteriorating the finger joints. Infections, although less common than the previous factors, can travel from other parts of the body and trigger pain, particularly when inflammation occurs. These are the three main factors which might be causing pain in your joints and leading to a feeling of weakness around this area.

3.1. Inflammatory Causes

Because joints are affected physiologically in conditions that are typically thought to be systemic, any doctor who deals with musculoskeletal complaints will be conversant with these types. The conclusions from your symptoms are often more critical than the findings from your sensitive and radiological tests (x-rays, MRI, CT scan), and the diagnosis and therapy protocols significantly rely on those conclusions. The immune system, working alone or in connection with the rest of the body, is at least partially responsible in such situations. The disease causes an increase in the cells in the synovial membrane's prospective area of development. The average number of synoviocytes per square millimeter will rise from two million to two million. This event results in synovial cell hyperplasia, a process that generates pannus. The disease causes new tissues to leak and destroy the joints, which has caused duplication of the small veins (venules) in 5-10 percent of the population.

While joint pain, damage, and weakness may occur as a result of chronic or excessive physical activity, it may also develop from a variety of other inflammatory and non-inflammatory causes. This section will focus on causes that mostly center on the inflammatory or immune response. Autoimmune, immune-mediated, inflammatory, and non-inflammatory joint conditions, syndromes, and diseases might result in discomfort, pathologies, and loss of function by causing damage to the joint. Rheumatoid arthritis is an example of an autoimmune condition in which symptoms and joint damage arise because the body's immune system undergoes an exacerbation.

3.2. Degenerative Causes

In the spine, osteoarthritis and loss of disc height (but also having the vertebra between the disc spaces push forward, or sublux into the disc) can cause an impingement on the nerves as they divide from the spinal cord and exit the spine known as stenosis. This decrease in the space where the nerves exit the spine is a key contributor to the pain and the potential nerve symptoms that result called radiculopathy or radiculitis. The compression is progressive, resulting generally in progressive weakness in addition to pain. Other degenerative conditions, usually in individuals of middle ages or older, that are capable of causing joint pain and stiffness and weakness include cervical spondylosis, carpal tunnel syndrome, and many of the other ways we can reduce nerve or muscle function implicated in muscle weakness discussed above.

Osteoarthritis is a common cause of many degenerative joint conditions. Osteoarthritis happens when there is a loss of cartilage in the joint. Because cartilage is a smooth, glistening lining at the ends of long bones that helps reduce friction and pain with normal joint use, once it's gone the joint can produce pain and crepitus (simple grind) as bone grinds against bone. The joint space becomes smaller, and cysts may form about the joint. The decreased joint space and myriad of cysts gives the surrounding bone an increased density on x-ray known as sclerosis, as well as bone overgrowth or bone spurs, known as osteophytes.

3.3. Infectious Causes

Infectious causes. Commonly, infections by various pathogens can target various joints in the body and affect the bones and the joint fluid, usually due to some prior infection and an unhealthy lifestyle. Normally, such infections result from a viral attack, though bacterial infections are also relatively common. Such infectious bacteria primarily represent the presence of a bacterium called Borrelia burgdorferi, which can be transmitted to other persons through tick bites or ticks. A number of viral infections have also been observed to be the main infectious cause of joint pain and weakness. Agents such as Togaviruses and Dengue have been observed to subsequently affect joint health and cause medical conditions called viral arthritis and Dengue virus-related joint pain. HIV, mumps, parvovirus, Hep A virus, and Hep B virus are the other major agents included in joint pain and weakness. Scientific research has recorded that viruses could directly attack the joint tissues or inflammatory conditions that can occur as a consequence of the immune response to clear these viral bodies out of the system and even signal pathways that can directly affect joint health. Some studies are also mentioning HIV prognosis through causing arthritis in patients and releasing toxins that can affect immune response factors and lead to inflammation in patients. The most common symptoms of infectious joint pain are usually seen to depend on the precise infectious activity's origin, severity, or the inflammation produced, but also the pathogen's type. However, indications such as joint pain, weakness, and a limited or restricted movement are commonly seen in most affected persons. Swelling and redness are also frequent signs, usually demonstrated as skin symptoms around the joint site of infection. Constitutional and systemic symptoms (such as lethargy, fever, and diarrhea) may occur in a variety of cases as well. The incidence of conditions, medications, and the immune health of all individuals involved in managing or interfering with the pathogens is considered as a prognosis and treatment option. Across all cases, joint diseases have been agreed upon as infectious agents. In reality, CNS infections usually require an MRI or lumbar puncture, whereas any unresponsiveness to antibiotic therapy may reject the use of IV antibiotics.

4. Symptoms of Joint Pain and Weakness

In general, joint pain and muscle weakness are considered distinct symptoms caused by fundamentally different mechanisms. The presence of both suggests weakness either within the muscles or the nerves designed to activate the muscle. When joint pain and muscle weakness coexist, most likely the problem is deep within the joint itself. Many people with joint pain may also have weakness, but the weakness is rarely as prominent as the pain. The most common symptoms experienced by individuals who seek medical attention for joint pain and muscle weakness in a particular region of the body include: The affected area exhibits a feeling of discomfort in the joint pain. Joints flare up and become swollen and warm to the touch.

Joint pain often produces a feeling of discomfort, a dull ache, or burning in the affected area. It can also produce stiffness, which makes it problematic to move the joint. Joint pain and muscle weakness can also induce weakness in other symptoms in the body, particularly the muscles of a particular region of the body. Imagine trying to bear weight on and use an arm or hand with joint pain. The pain in the joint is likely to make the surrounding muscles weaker than usual. People often hold limbs with joint pain still to avoid pain because movement tends to aggravate the existing discomfort. The lack of movement may induce the limb to develop weakness from disuse. The end result is muscle atrophy, which is a general term for muscle loss.

Signs of Joint Weakness: Typically, the muscles responsible for indirect or circumducting hip or joint movement weaken first. After that, the muscles in the upper part of the trunk on the same side start to weaken. Individuals may become aware that something is wrong when they feel discomfort while getting up from a sitting position. Over time, leg weakness develops.

The signs and symptoms of joint disease vary depending on the type of joint disease causing them. For many individuals living with joint diseases, the symptoms come and go and are usually more severe in the early morning. Even slight movement can cause discomfort and pain, but the joint improves and the pain subsides as they move. For others, the leg muscles and joints become weaker and stiffer over time. An individual who is not only in pain but also weak is likely to have a limp while walking or may alter their walking to keep the affected joint mobile. Low-level joint weakness can manifest, for example, in simple daily tasks such as using the fingers to unscrew a bolt from a bottle or opening a lid.

Pain and stiffness, frequently accompanied by swelling and weakness, can occur in joints as a result of either underlying diseases or accidental injury. It is found to be a common cause of joint pain and weakness. The most common types of joint diseases that cause joint pain and weakness include rheumatoid arthritis (RA), lupus, and osteoarthritis. While RA and lupus affect younger individuals, the incidence of these diseases increases with age.

1. Atypical symptoms Atypical symptoms of joint pain and weakness do occur, although less frequently. Joint pain may sometimes be atypical in its presentation or location; it may occur especially at night when a person is at rest. Joint pain is not thought to be occurring in that part of the body that is adjoining the affected bone joint that has a problem. Some unusual or atypical causes of joint pain include: ovary pain that may feel like hip, back, or sometimes leg pain, so the disease can occur up inside of the hip area colorectal cancer, tenderness near the upper outer edges of the hip bone may be related to ovarian cancer, hemiparesis-weakness on one side of the body, many times sudden weakness may have a pattern of the stroke-like clinical syndrome, cluster of weakness can result in leg dragging – sciatic nerve syndrome, other causes of gait disturbance, changes in walking, or weakness or leg dragging. In some cases, tests that are designed to reproduce the person's pain are negative. This is generally because the test may not be sensitive enough and the patient may not be in so much of acute distress to reproduce their pain. Other atypical findings include a joint that has minimal swelling (spinal stenosis); irritability and mental status changes (CNS causes); recent IV drug use, malignancy, liver disease, or other immuno-suppressing condition. The presence of a constitutional symptom, the patient's foot is cold but they feel it is hot, history of a previous fracture, severe night pain in a patient that is under 18, and unexplained high fevers are "red flags" and

should prompt the clinician to do thorough work up and urgent imaging.

Identifying common symptoms can help diagnose the patient in a better way, but atypical symptoms can make diagnosis more challenging.

Atypical signs of joint pain and weakness

5. Diagnosis of Joint Pain and Weakness

A long, thin, hollow needle is often utilized to gather a microscopic sample of liquid from inside a swollen joint. This is generally accomplished using fluoroscopic radiology or an ultrasound to help the doctor know exactly where to insert the needle. In this procedure, a needle is utilized to take a tiny amount of liquid from a joint. Alleviating pain and stiffness in the joint relieve symptoms such as pain, inflammation, and swelling. The doctor sends the fluid to a laboratory to be examined for the presence of crystals and/or microorganisms. A negative or positive result can be used to indicate the presence of illness.

Imaging methods for joints might include the following: - Radiographs, also known as x-rays (X-rays) - Ultrasonography or MRI (magnetic resonance imaging) (ultrasound) - Computerized tomography (CT scan) - Joint aspiration for synovial fluid testing - Joint fluid examination

Doctors who evaluate joint pain and weakness perform a physical examination and frequently request imaging tests and blood work. A physical assessment is performed to evaluate the patient's physical health. Your doctor may check your heart, lungs, and reflexes, as well as monitor your joint range of motion and sensation. Blood tests such as a complete blood count (CBC), erythrocyte sedimentation rate (ESR), rheumatoid factor, C-reactive protein (CRP), and creatine kinase surface antigens are frequently requested. Other tests can also be requested.

Advanced imaging methods are frequently used to see the inside of joints and the tissues that surround them. These tests may also help doctors see whether an injury or illness is present, as well as how serious it may be. Many of these tests are performed in a hospital's radiology (X-ray) department.

5.1. Physical Examination

The physical examination is much more rewarding for the clinician. The muscles and all of the nerves that innervate them can generally be separated into the cephalic and caudal halves. There are exceptions, but if the suprascapular nerve is affected, the muscles it innervates are proximal or more cephalic than muscles supplied by nerves coming from the level of C5. Where the nerve is entrapped affects more muscles than the particular nerve. Joints are evaluated for abnormal changes in mobility, both passively and actively. The muscles moving the joint are then tested in a skull-to-face manner, meaning that the proximal muscles are tested first. This gives a quick assessment of whether the problem is mostly proximal (such as a pinched nerve in the neck) or something more peripheral.

The first step in evaluating joint pain and weakness is a careful history and physical examination. There are a number of concerns of the history and special aspects of the physical examination that facilitate the diagnosis. The site of the pain is a clue to the diagnosis, as is radiation or variation with neck flexion or extension in a patient with arm pain. Some patients have combinations of upper and lower motor neuron findings, differentiated by signs of a lesion in the head (pretty rare). In general, imaging studies are not particularly helpful with a patient who has been seen for treatment peripherally. They are performed initially if there is pain that might indicate the need for surgery, a "red flag" in the history, or if things are not getting better with treatment.

5.2. Imaging Techniques

While the above imaging tools are used to observe the structure of the bone and surrounding tissues and incapacity, while it does not uncover the active state of the disease or the hidden damage within the tissues. As part of radiology, nuclear medicine imaging tools including the technetium 99m bone scan and three-phase bone scintigraphy are used for imaging the bone in search of tumors and infections as well as the spread of cancer into the bone, such as to determine whether joint pain is due to bone infection, bursitis, cellulitis, or septic arthritis. The bone scan will distinguish between the old and the new injury and can detect stress fractures at a much earlier time compared to an X-ray. A diagnostic ultrasound is another useful tool that helps examine injuries in the muscles, ligament, cartilage, and tendons which are often the causes of joint pain. It is fast and gives instant images and can also differentiate between whether the swelling or pain is due to the trapped nerve or whether it is the worse symptoms that spreading from the joint so that appropriate treatment can be given.

Imaging techniques are used to identify and understand joint pain or weakness that is often associated with different types of arthritis. An X-ray is often the first imaging modality to be tried and may show narrowing of the spaces between two bones of the joints, changes in the bone itself, and the formation of new bone. However, X-rays are only useful when the condition has progressed or progressed quite a bit. Magnetic resonance imaging (MRI) and CT (computed tomography) scan are also employed to show changes in the bones and the surrounding ligaments and tendons in greater detail than an X-ray. While CT is usually combined with myelography in order to visualize the soft tissues, MRI is considered the best imaging tool for detecting the early damage to the bone cartilage, the formation of cysts, and changes in synovium, and the ligament, and the capsule.

5.3. Laboratory Tests

Lactate, pyruvate, and synovial fluid glucose are commonly tested. Lactic acid level, typically 10%-20% of the blood value, is much lower than that in serum due to its rapid utilization for cellular energy inside chondrocytes. The arthrocentesis sample is also tested for the presence of blood. The serum uric acid level is tested for diagnosing gout and pseudogout. Serum rheumatoid factor (RF), anti-nuclear antibody (ANA), anti-double-stranded DNA (anti-dsDNA) to aid in diagnosing systemic lupus erythematosus (SLE), anti-DNA, anti-centromere, anti-Sjogren's syndrome, anti-SS-A, and anti-SS-B are also tested when necessary. Serum electrolyte levels and tests for calcium, alkaline phosphatase, hepatic, and renal function are used to identify calcium pyrophosphate dihydrate deposition and other related conditions. Erythrocyte sedimentation rate (ESR) and C-reactive protein (CRP) can also help in diagnosis, while the diagnosis of culture-positive infection can be performed with synovial fluid bacterial culture.

Laboratory tests are significant in confirming a diagnosis if the patient is experiencing any other symptoms in addition to joint pain and weakness. These tests augment physical examinations and radiographic results. Arthrocentesis samples are examined for analysis. Laboratory tests include the complete blood count (CBC), including white blood cell (WBC) count, red blood cell (RBC) count, hemoglobin (Hb), hematocrit (Hct), and platelet count. Arthrocentesis may show leukocytosis, erythrocytosis, monocytosis, and changes indicative of rheumatic diseases.

However, some normal aspirates as well as pathological aspirates may be obtained, depending on the stage of abnormality and underlying disease process. Individuals receiving anticoagulants or those who have bleeding disorders can cause a barrier to obtaining the sample.

6. Treatment Options

4. Osteotomy This operation, appropriate for healthy young adult patients who are unhappy with low demand levels and Emmett regularly injured, changes the sides of the bones in the knee. This moves your weight from the inside to the outside of your knee.

3. Debridement The destruction of the ends of the bones due to inflammation. This can generally be done with arthroscopy, or an open type of operation performed by the patient.

2. Arthrodesis The diseased part must be attached together to form a new joint.

1. Arthroscopy Arthroscopic surgery is used to diagnose and repair joint problems that affect joint pain and stiffness.

Surgery may be necessary in some cases for joint pain and weakness. Your physician may recommend damage repair, such as torn ligaments, meniscus, or other joint injuries. Joint replacement surgery may also be recommended to repair any large joint (knee, hip, elbow, etc.). Surgery of joints includes:

4. Medications Some of these include over-the-counter and/or prescription-strength NSAIDs, such as Ibuprofen, Naproxen, Meloxicam, or Diclofenac to diminish inflammation and pain, as well as Tylenol to alleviate pain. Tramadol and some narcotics can aid in modulation and

abatement of pain that can result in improvement in RA or require opioids with strong medications.

3. Injections Steroids and/or Hyaluronic Acid Injections. These two types of injections help reduce inflammation causing joint pain and weakness.

2. Occupational Therapy The physical therapy aids in coping with the day-to-day requirement of joint pain and weakness is referred to as occupational therapy.

1. Physical Therapy This treatment plan includes specific movements to strengthen and mobilize the affected joint, muscle groups, or tendons. Your therapist might have you engage in walking, running, or swimming. Physical therapy can help you increase your range of motion, decrease pain, and improve your strength in the area. This therapy may involve using training equipment like treadmills and weight machines. Your therapist may choose manual therapy to apply a force to your muscles and perform a postural reeducation program to retrain the way the muscles coordinate.

The treatment for your joint pain and weakness is more accessible to determine with the correct diagnosis. You may need different strategies for different causes. For example, your osteoarthritis might benefit more from motion-based therapy, while a rheumatoid arthritis diagnosis may involve different types of medication that are priced into your insurance policy. Some therapy types recommended for your joint pain and weakness are:

6.1. Medications

To effectively treat joint pain and weakness, the best pain management approach considers the underlying cause as well as related symptoms. Relieving pain in the joints may also help to maintain or increase an individual's quality of life. Treatment options are conservative to start, moving to surgery when it has been decided that non-invasive treatment isn't effective. According to your diagnosis, your healthcare team may use one or more options. Some people find relief from over-the-counter (OTC) medications such as pain relievers and NSAIDs. If they didn't help, a doctor may recommend some combination of long-term medication, ongoing physical therapy, heat or cold therapy, splints, joint braces, supportive footwear, taping, assistive devices, regular exercise, foam rolling, and even surgery.

Treatment for Joint Pain and Weakness

- Analgesics: A mild pain reliever such as aspirin, acetaminophen, or an opiate. - Nonsteroidal anti-inflammatory drugs (NSAIDs): Common over-the-counter NSAIDs include aspirin, ibuprofen, and naproxen. - Corticosteroids: A strong anti-inflammatory taken by mouth, by injection, or applied topically (to the skin). - Other drugs: A lot of different drugs may be used in combination with others to treat different symptoms. For symptoms related to joint pain and weakness, medication may also reduce inflammation or slow down the progression of autoimmune diseases like rheumatoid arthritis.

For those with chronic joint pain or weakness, medications can be part of managing your condition. A doctor can talk to you about the reason for your pain, and they may suggest what to use for joint pain. They are typically sorted by the impact they have on the body (opiates like codeine are stronger than aspirin, for example), as well as by whether or not they could lead to misuse. Common medications for joint pain include:

6.2. Physical Therapy

An exercise program consisting of flexibility and strengthening exercises is important. Strengthening exercises typically focus on muscle groups that provide dynamic support at the joint. For example, a person with hip instability may need to participate in an exercise program that is heavy in adductor and core exercises. Muscle strengthening is also important and should focus on retraining muscles that stabilize the knee, hip, and other joints so that proper movement patterns are maintained when lifting, sitting, walking, or participating in activities of daily living. Proper form, movement, and lifting techniques are important. Rehabilitation programs may also focus on less activity-specific training programs, such as core strengthening or multipoint exercises, if they are a contributing factor to joint pain. Other athletic-type exercises may include balance and plyometrics. In addition to passive interventions, several therapeutic modalities and exercises may be used to improve physical function.

Because joint pain and weakness are often due to complex pathology, the treatment of joint pain often includes a focus on several contributing factors together. Physical therapists are often involved in the treatment and management of this condition. Physical therapy treatments may include physical modalities such as ice, heat, or ultrasound, manual therapy or massage to improve joint function and range of motion, as well as exercises such as stretching and resistance programs. Quadriceps exercises are often used to improve the strength of the knee extensor muscles. A slow-speed resistance program has also been shown in research studies to be beneficial for pain relief and strength improvement in people with lower-extremity injuries.

6.3. Surgical Interventions

In the Netherlands, joint replacement in end-stage knee or hip osteoarthritis is an effective and advisable treatment option. The endoprosthesis provides the patient with a painless joint, thereby improving the patient's quality of life. For a successful long-term follow-up, patients are advised to follow activity and weight prescriptions. Blood supply and support in bone structure are important to the successful outcome of the prosthesis. In arthroscopy, the doctor makes several small incisions around the joint and inserts rubber tubes, called cannulas, to keep the joint open and in good view. The doctor then inserts the arthroscope, which is about the size of a pencil. Patients usually go home the same day or after one night in the hospital. After surgery, patients will be shown exercises that will help strengthen the joint. They also may be referred to a physical therapist. Total hip and knee replacement procedures are the most invasive of these options, and they are the most effective. After joint replacement, a patient can lead a more normal and less painful life, though the joint may never feel exactly the same as before it was damaged.

Acute care. Surgical interventions. Surgery is considered an option for individuals with severe joint-related disorders. Common pathologies managed operatively include arthrosis of the knee and hip and severe shoulder and elbow conditions. Potential surgical interventions include: • Total joint replacement • Hemiartroplasty • Joint resurfacing • Arthroplastic surgery • Arthroscopic surgery

7. Preventive Measures

7.1. Lifestyle Changes

7.2. Exercise and Stretching

8. Complications of Untreated Joint Pain and Weakness

Traumatic causes can lead to further injury, scarring, or other sequelae. Neglecting joint pain and weakness is expected to result in future joint problems that may lead to replacements or other interventions. The good news is that these complications can typically be avoided by early management of joint problems. Learning more about muscles and joints can help us better understand what and why certain aspects cause joint pain and weakness. The more we understand this, the better we can manage and even educate others on how to live a healthier lifestyle.

Joint pain and various joint diseases can be challenging. Without proper education and prompt attention, joint pain can severely affect your quality of life and prevent normal daily activities. If left untreated, joint pain can lead to the following complications: limb weakness can decrease your ability to withstand normal forces, resulting in a downward spiral into inactivity and increased atrophy, weakness, and pain. Soft or periarticular tissue disorders, as well as muscle weakness or imbalance, can place further strain on the joint, leading to further dysfunction and pain. Flares may lead to learned fear, phobia, and potential avoidance of physical activity. This can result in reduced ranges of motion, muscle stiffness, further weakness, and even atrophy if the symptoms persist long enough.

9. Future Research and Developments

One such research question is to understand the symptoms of muscle pain as a cause of secondary musculoskeletal pain and the role of peripheral sensory receptors in generating the pain. The development of pain tests to identify relevant subgroups of patients continues to be a strong research area. In addition, myalgia research often contributes to drugs that are first used by rheumatology. The present adult measures and interventions identify relief through physical pathways in mid-age populations, including those used in cancer populations, but are not adult neuromodulation. The new adult measures and interventions likely to be identified in the future are not likely to be adult neuromodulation. Neuromodulation will be responsible for the development of methods of identifying less interference with brain functional magnetic resonance imaging and reducing neuromodulation use in mid-aged populations.

Several areas of research are developing in the area of joint pain and weakness. New treatments for people with osteoarthritis and musculoskeletal conditions are likely to be an important part of the musculoskeletal agenda, such as mesenchymal stem cells, which have already undergone a number of high-quality trials. If sufficiently effective and economic treatments are shown, traction may help prevent the need for extensive joint replacement. Other areas of potential development include muscle-strengthening exercises to reduce the rate of pain development, new, more accurate and non-invasive diagnostic technologies, such as blood tests to predict a future joint replacement in someone with early knee pain, and preventive strategies that help those people whose x-rays are consistent with a musculoskeletal condition develop symptoms at a reduced rate.

10. Conclusion

It can be concluded that joint pain and weakness and their consequences should be known to a joint and that this understanding should influence the clinical diagnosis and treatment involving joints. To understand the causes, one should be aware of the anatomic distribution and physiology. The determination of the following of the joint pain and joint weaknesses at an early stage is the touchstone for any disease, and the earlier the better. The appropriate duration of the treatment with minimum invasiveness is the motto. Prevention is always better than cure for a joint. It may not be very serious in the earlier stages but it initiated at someone's juncture. That will be a minor problem to go for an extended period. It is easier to explore before a complete joint physiologies complete failure. Hence, one should be aware of such problems in the particular body and seek doctors' advice accordingly.

A joint is a connecting part of two or more bones, which is directly related to the human body's movement. In such a case, the joint's importance becomes paramount. To understand joint pain and weakness to the highest extent, it is important to understand the anatomy of the joint. It is also important to have knowledge of the different parts related to a joint and the whole joint. Joint pain and joint weakness are drivers in certain diseases and also affect body movements. Joint pain and weakness are important factors that affect arthritis and rheumatism in people around the world. Joint pain and weakness in a joint are concerned with soft tissues and hard tissues such as cartilage, tendons, and bone. Many diseases like OA, RA, gout, are a few of the joint pain diseases which are related to arthritis and their associated diseases.

Understanding the Relationship Between Joint Pain and Weakness: 7 Conditions and Treatment Strategies

1. Introduction

In this guide, we'll walk you through seven conditions that might cause joint pain and weakness and break down the various treatment strategies you might consider as you work to recover. Because joint weakness and joint pain so often go hand-in-hand, many of the conditions that might contribute to one will also contribute to the other. Hemochromatosis, a genetic disorder, can lead to both joint pain and muscle weakness. One of its hallmarks is potential effects on the endocrine system, which could lead to symptoms that mirror arthritis and other joint pain conditions. Let's take a closer look at seven causes of joint weakness that could also result in joint damage.

Joint pain and weakness are often felt together, which isn't terribly surprising. After all, both are symptoms of a certain degree of muscle weakness. When your muscles, including the ones that support your joints, aren't functioning as well as they should, you're apt to feel joint pain and weakness. A variety of factors can cause weak muscles in your body. Injury and degenerative bone or nerve conditions can cause muscle weakness and joint damage at the same time. Meanwhile, everything from nutritional deficiencies to fungal infections can lead to muscle weakness and joint problems. While the precise nature of the relationship between joint pain and weakness can change on a case-to-case basis (and depend on the root cause), knowing your options for relief and recovery can be empowering.

1.1. Definition and Overview of Joint Pain and Weakness

Weakness, conversely, may also happen for several reasons. It includes illness, depression, pain, or fatigue. For all individuals, lack of strength can have a major influence on the quality of life and the capacity to carry out everyday tasks. Knowledge on disability and muscular weakness is important as it impacts the individual's capacity to function normally, to undergo physical treatment, and allows the coordination to be affected. Over the course of their life, people may experience joint pain and/or weakness at different points. In certain instances, patients can experience joint pain and weakness at the same time. Although the problems may not be connected in these circumstances, it is often important as both are potential signs of a single disease.

Joint pain is a common condition affecting individuals of all ages. It can be mild, causing slight discomfort, or severe, resulting in limited or decreased function of the affected joint. Joint pain may also range from being acute, lasting anywhere from a few hours or days, to chronic, persisting for periods longer than three months. The pain experienced may be localized, resulting only in discomfort on movement or palpation of one part of the joint, or widespread, leading to discomfort in the surrounding joints or muscles. Joint pain tends to increase with age and affects around one-third of the adult population, with more frequent incidence in women than men. Lastly, joint pain is not associated with any specific gender, though it affects the left and right sides of the body.

1.2. Significance of Understanding the Relationship

The possibility that pain reduces volitional muscle activation undermines the results of strength tests and promotes gait changes or stops people with poor outcomes engaging in standard therapy. When pain reduction emerges independently of strength change, is seen across tasks and delays, including measurements that cannot be influenced by mental distraction or conscious effort, and moderates outcome irrespective of pain improvement, the clinical significance should be self-evident. Numerous additional factors modulate how muscle activity can be inferred from measures of joint torque, which can be seen in both symptomatic tendinopathy and knee osteoarthritis. It is therefore also important to emphasize the need for strength co-creating interventions to target the issue directly. Various physical examination observations suggest that changes in movement, co-contraction, strength, and muscle timing can be evinced in one condition but not the other, but whether these are cause or effect is less clear.

Given the recognition that some patients seek care for joint symptoms before pain becomes measurable, understanding the relationship between joint pain and weakness could be of benefit to patients, providers, and investigators. While it is accepted that disability across multiple dimensions is common in OA, multiple non-pharmacological interventions target weaknesses around painful joints, generally on the pretext that the muscle weakness present either causes or amplifies joint symptoms. Recognizing that distal inhibitors (such as muscle weakness) can decrease the efficacy of volitional activities, including strength testing tasks, generalization to clinical and research settings necessitates a valid methodology to stratify patients on this attribute as a function of their underlying task-specific weakness.

2. Conditions That Cause Joint Pain and Weakness

One of the most common conditions in old ages is osteoarthritis. This type of arthritis is an articular cartilage research arising from age-related, traumatic, or mechanical environmental factors. Many signs and symptoms have been linked to the disease, including morning stiffness, joint crepitation, and decreased joint or nearby musculatures strength and weakness. In osteoarthritis, joint weakness is an unpleasant and common experience. Rheumatoid arthritis is an autoimmune disease characterized by the destruction of the joints. As in osteoarthritis, symptoms of rheumatoid arthritis are fatigue, weakness, and pain that can be seen on both sides of the body equally. Fibromyalgia is involved in soft tissue, poor sleep, increased sensitivity to pain, and muscular fatigue. Like all the aforementioned conditions, fibromyalgia also presents fatigue, weakness, and pain, particularly if traumatic exposure is considered. In observing the 243 patients with either osteoarthritis or fibromyalgia, it has been revealed that they mostly complain of pain and weakness.

Although the joints and muscles have different pathophysiological systems, some factors affect both parts. It isn't easy to find a common explanation for this situation. However, some professionals have listed several conditions that can lead to both joint weakness and pain. In this article, we focused on these classes, which are osteoarthritis, rheumatoid arthritis, fibromyalgia, lupus, bursitis, tendonitis, and osteoporosis. It is no secret that osteoporosis both weakens the bones and leads to joint fractures. In arthritis, inflammations in the bones may lead to joint weakening. In bursitis, the symptoms of the condition progress to a point that weakens the muscle tone that has the potential to lead to joint weakness.

2.1. 1. Osteoarthritis

During the development of osteoarthritis, joint injuries can cause greater harm. Arthritis can lead to decreased physical mobility and exercise capacity. However, it should not cause significant pain or disability. Pain can be caused by a reduction in motor strength in close or decompensated muscles, resulting in joint instability, injury to the joint, and injury to the surrounding muscles and soft tissues. Due to the emotional stress associated with OA, cognitive and mood disturbances are common when experiencing long-term joint pain and weakness. This can lead to panic attacks and decreased concentration. It is often important to consult a mental health professional to ensure optimal psychiatric attention, counseling, or psychotherapy as part of a comprehensive treatment program. Information about prognosis and treatment should be provided openly. If possible, start planning for treatment. Treating the acute phase should be a priority, focusing on reducing pain and instability and achieving the therapeutic goals mentioned above. All of this should improve the patient's response to discomfort and promote constructive levels of work, entertainment, and stamina.

Osteoarthritis (OA) is the most common diagnosis that causes joint pain and weakness. Osteoarthritis can affect any joint; it is common in the knees, back, and hips. Symptoms of osteoarthritis usually include pain, stiffness, joint tenderness, reduced range of motion, and pain during workouts. Some activities can increase the risk of developing osteoarthritis, including joint injuries. Many joint injuries cause more cartilage damage than they treat. Other accidents, such as muscle injuries, fractures, and dislocations, can also increase the risk of arthritis.

RA attacks the knees or other joints directly through several mechanisms: Synovitis: The synovium is tissue inside the knees that provides nutrients and components to help lubricate the knee joint. In RA, the synovium gets inflamed, which can cause swelling and may lead to pain when the swelling triggers pain-sensing nerves. Local muscle around the knees can get affected directly by the inflammatory process, which can interfere with muscles' ability to help stabilize the knee joint (leading to weakness). In RA, the immune system creates antibodies. In other words, the body makes specific proteins that mistakenly attack other parts of the body. In about 70% of cases, the immune system creates and releases anti-citrullinated protein antibodies (ACPAs). Inflammatory processes go through bodies where the immune system creates chemicals that promote inflammation. Cell-mediated immunity: Immune cells called T-cells may also slow down the rate at which muscle tissues can recover in RA. Muscle tissue of the thigh gets affected in people with RA too. One trial showed that muscle strength and performance measured after exercise (maximum voluntary isometric contraction (MVIC) torque and muscle power) was lower in thigh muscles of people with RA compared to people who do not have RA. Those authors concluded that increased muscle inflammation due to RA may decrease muscle performance.

Rheumatoid arthritis (RA) is an autoimmune condition. This means the immune system mistakenly attacks the body, which can affect more than just joint health. Although RA is often associated with the hands, it can affect other joints, such as the knees. An estimated 87-89% of people with RA may experience weakness in and around the knees, while other joints can be affected. The symptoms of a proactive or flare-up of RA may include knee weakness along with swelling, pain, and stiffness. During a flare-up, the body goes through periods where the immune system mistakenly sends chemicals and cells to attack foreign substances that don't exist around the joint that is being attacked. The symptoms experienced during an RA flare-up can be triggered by factors that raise inflammation and/or the immune system getting "over-activated."

Rheumatoid Arthritis

2.3. 3. Fibromyalgia

As this is an inflammatory or pathologies report, it will focus on an in-depth look at fibromyalgia and the potential condition-specific problems surrounding joint pain in the context of a connective tissue disorder or some of the coexisting symptoms of the disease tied to daily activity dysfunction. Chronic pain can change the way that the body functions with use and subsequently decrease the pain threshold in the presence of any load applied, consequently increasing the pain experienced and setting up the individual for a perpetual pain cycle. Additionally, strength and, for that matter, any muscle improvements may plateau or manifest as negative strength gains in some instances. This could also negatively alter the way in which the body co-contracts in anticipation of joint pain for maintenance of joint integrity. Although little is understood about the relationship, abnormalities in the joint/autoimmune disorders of varying makeups have been reported in many wider fibromyalgia studies.

Fibromyalgia is an incredibly painful and chronic musculoskeletal condition causing fatigue and stiffness, accompanied by "tender points," which can cause pain with applied pressure. An understanding of fibromyalgia and the symptoms associated with the disease will also be included to gain a clearer picture of how the coexisting symptoms of growth pain and weakness due to other potential conditions could further decrease functional status and daily performance. A pathophysiological description of the condition will also be included in an attempt to better understand how symptoms unique to the pathology could result in decreased day to day function and joint-related complaints. Fibromyalgia is characterized by widespread pain and is often accompanied by fatigue and difficulty sleeping. The symptoms can mimic other conditions such as chronic fatigue syndrome and, as such, it is difficult to unequivocally say what the true incidence rate of fibromyalgia in the world is.

Weakness associated with lupus is often felt symmetrically - it can be physically measured on opposite sides of the body, like in the shoulder girdles or thighs. People with lupus have reported having a lot of difficulty using stairs as a result of the proximal muscle weakness in the legs. Some people with lupus have also been found to have low levels of insulin-like growth factor-1 in the blood. This growth hormone signals the body to keep skin, muscle, and bone well-maintained, and lower levels of insulin-like growth factor-1 have been associated with lower grip strength and dry grip strength in people with lupus. Certain nerve problems are due to small fiber neuropathy, which is different from the more clinical carpal tunnel or ulnar neuropathies we mentioned above. This problem with the small nerve fibers is easily identified using a skin biopsy prefix - one of those many procedures.

Lupus isn't simply about the immune system attacking the body. There are different kinds of lupus with different concerns, symptoms, and immunological markers. The ANA blood test is not very specific for lupus, so errors in the literature in summarizing lupus information are common. Lupus is an autoimmune disease where the body attacks itself, causing widespread inflammation and tissue damage. It can cause the skin, joints, kidneys, blood cells, and other systems of the body to become inflamed. There are different types of lupus. The most common form of lupus, and the form that most people are referring to when they say "lupus," is Systemic Lupus Erythematosus (SLE).

This form can affect any part of the body. People with lupus are more likely to have malaise, muscle pain, fever, and weakness.

2.5. 5. Osteoporosis

Some cases of osteoporosis are asymptomatic, meaning that no overt symptoms are often observed. Nevertheless, osteoporosis can result in a number of symptoms directly related to the bones. For example, patients may notice that over time, they have lost height or that their posture has changed; stooping or bending forward due to fracture of the vertebra. They may also notice pain in the back and pain radiating down the back, gasping for breath when bending forward. In other instances, osteoporosis having gone undiagnosed until a fracture in the wrist, hip, or spine revealed its presence. In the event of a fracture, pain and an accompanying weakness may be pronounced, inhibiting mobility and overall quality of life. Osteoporosis care commonly places a focus on working in a prophylactic manner to prevent falls and fractures. Doing so is based around a whole-of-life strategy by ensuring that there are enough minerals in a good, balanced diet throughout the different life stages. It is not just "drinking more milk"!

A significant factor to consider when addressing joint pain and weakness is bone health. After all, bone deterioration can result in a decrease in bone density, leaving the structure of the joint supported by increasingly weak bones. This aspect of joint pain and weakness is particularly problematic when osteoporosis comes into play, as this condition already results in a decrease in bone mineral density. Osteoporosis is often associated with the fracture of bones in areas such as the hip, spine, and wrist, injuries which often result in chronic pain, weakness, and an increase in the risk of arthritis in these areas.

Osteoporosis as a cause of joint pain and weakness

2.6. 6. Bursitis

The pain of bursitis often starts mildly and can be explained away as the result of overworking the joint. Symptoms of joint pain associated with bursitis can include stiffness, the loss of ability to move the affected part of the body normally due to pain, and local swelling. Large joints like the shoulder, hip, and knee may appear warm to touch. Bursitis differs from arthritis because joint stiffness present in bursitis usually occurs in the morning but eases during the day. There may also be an increase in discomfort if the person stays in one position for a prolonged period. Tenderness and achiness of the joint that can radiate into the upper and middle back may also accompany the pain. Pain from bursitis can make sleeping on the side of the shoulder or hip uncomfortable. The pain becomes more severe if the affected part is moved or pressed, making daily activities a challenge. Discerning the reason for weakness and then treating the underlying problem can help you find relief from joint pain.

Our joints have many components, which means joint pain may have different origins. Sometimes, problems begin when the bursae become inflamed through overuse or repetitive stress from daily activities, leading to a condition known as bursitis. This inflammation of the bursa sacs in the shoulder, elbow, hip, or knee typically causes pain, particularly in the shoulder or hip, as the bursae are in close proximity to these body parts. The joint pain associated with bursitis may also include weakness, leading to symptoms such as dragging the foot or locking or jamming in position when bending a limb. Bursitis may be associated with a sudden injury or trauma, such as a fall or blow to the body. For many people, repetitive motion or overuse causes the condition. Hip bursitis is often misdiagnosed as trochanteric bursitis, which is pain from the curve of the hip bone that can travel down the side of the leg. However, the main type of bursitis linked to the hip is iliopectineal bursitis, which is the inflammation of a pelvic bursa rather than a hip bursa.

Tendonitis contributes to joint pain and weakness since the tendons involved, while thick, aren't meant to withstand extreme forces. Consequently, tendonitis will begin to break down the tendons, creating a weaker joint area. As tendonitis continues to decline, the pain results from a decrease in movement or overall flexibility. Often, tendonitis—typically referred to as golfer's elbow, tennis elbow, or swimmer's shoulder—isn't referred to by the term tendonitis because it refers to a particular area of the body. Tendonitis has specific qualities solely expressing itself in the tendons of the body. Spurs of relative bone can break off of the joint region over time and come to rest in the tendons, leading to pain and potential tears. That tear in the tendon leads mainly to reduced mobility and pain in the weak joint.

Those who complain about pain and weakness in their joints could be suffering from tendonitis. It affects the tissue that connects the muscles to the bones and usually occurs because of repetitive activity, overuse, or a minor or major injury. The condition can affect any part of the body where large, weight-bearing tendons are present, causing significant pain and other symptoms. Only a medical professional will be able to diagnose tendonitis accurately, feeling the problem area on the body and perhaps conducting an MRI or X-ray to see exactly what's causing the pain. Remedies usually start with conservative measures such as rest, ice, or a support brace. Steroid injections and surgery can sometimes be needed.

3. Common Treatment Strategies

Surgical intervention: Patients with weakened muscles and pain or severe pain secondary to a mechanical concern may require surgery. Weakening and stretching of an injured or weakened muscle is not recommended.

Nutritional supplements: Calcium, vitamin D, or glucosamine/chondroitin supplements do not repair weakened muscles or painful joints, but in some people, they may provide coverage.

Physical therapy and exercise: Physicians often refer patients for physical therapy to improve flexibility, strengthen the muscles around the affected area, and improve posture and functions.

Prior to starting these treatments for joint pain or weakness, consult online references and talk to your doctor about the drugs that may benefit you. Medications taken specifically to address pain and muscle weakness are termed "chemical throws." Most often, these are in the form of nonsteroidal anti-inflammatory drugs (NSAIDs), acetaminophen, and weak opiate medications. Topical anti-inflammatory substances, such as diclofenac, salicylates, or capsaicin, can also decrease muscle and joint pain. In conjunction with physical treatments, medications that are less directly pain-related can be used.

Lifestyle modification: Patients should avoid overuse and incorporate regular rest in daily activities. Patients may need to make adjustments at work or at home to relieve excessive stress on weakened painful joints or muscles. Assist devices, weight loss, and avoidance of excessive tension can all be advantageous. Other pain and/or weakness-relieving treatments can also help to ensure the success of conservative treatments, the healthy use of symptomatic joints, and the maintenance of muscle strength in those who respond to pain and weakness treatments.

Joint pain and weakness typically require a multifaceted treatment approach. In patients with associated comorbidities and multiple joint pain or weakness problems, the ideal treatment may alter standard treatment options to maximize safety and pain relief. Treatment options may occur concurrently during pain or weakness treatment.

3.1. 1. Medications

Analgesics reduce pain but not inflammation. Anesthetics prevent pain by causing a numbing sensation. Our experience is that they aren't the most effective in relieving pain and creating functional improvements; as the sole needle on the haystack, so to speak, symptoms will persist. Many patients use medications to dampen the immune response, such as corticosteroids and non-steroidal anti-inflammatory drugs, to relieve joint pain. Trying different medications and approaches with a recognized specialist is often the best course of action to relieve pain and limited physical function. Non-steroidal anti-inflammatory drugs are commonly known to help reduce the pain of inflammation, and its scientific evidence is consistent with its popularity. Recognize that non-steroidal anti-inflammatory drugs work for some people, but not to everyone, so keep this in mind if you don't experience relief while taking this medicine.

Medications offer several options for dealing with joint pain and accompanying weakness. While medication tends to address the symptoms of joint-related conditions rather than the causes of pain and/or weakness, the former might offer temporary relief and improve mobility while waiting for the latter to kick in. There are several types of medications that might help alleviate joint pain and weakness. In general, medications work either by interfering with the body's pain signals, subduing its immune response, or influencing the processes that are linked with its onset, like metabolism, or preventing joint degradation by addressing the underlying cause. However, their mechanisms of action can overlap and are often not entirely known, especially in the conditions listed below. Because the management of pain and weakness can vary for each patient, pharmacological options are sometimes a matter of trial and error—or preference.

3.2. 2. Physical Therapy and Exercise

Exercise and physical therapy offer numerous advantages for people with joint pain and muscle weakness, including improved joint mobilization, joint lubrication, muscle strength, muscle endurance, cardiopulmonary function, bone deposition, lymphatic flow/immunity, and lessening of stress on the inflamed tissues. This enables you to achieve more in your day-to-day lifestyle, recreation, and vocation. Regrettably, most of these beneficial physiological effects become diminished if you don't incorporate these exercises at least three times a week or more, and long-term throughout one's life. In the presence of severe joint effusion, meniscus tear, or atrophy, physical intervention in the form of joint aspiration or small electric currents could help improve the scope of motion. E-stim, in particular, has been demonstrated to be effective in ameliorating the pain and quadriceps atrophy associated with arthritis.

Exercise, in particular supervised physical therapy, plays a pivotal role in the management of joint pain and weakness. Resistance training improves muscle strength, while flexibility exercises have been demonstrated to increase range of motion around affected joints. Those with advanced or brittle bones may require adjustments or gentle handling by their therapist. Supervised physical activity for arthritis is demonstrated to be more beneficial than education alone. After completing physical therapy, these exercises should become part of your regular routine. Certain people with knee pain might potentially benefit from a later start to exercises, particularly if arthritis symptoms and normal motion are managed.

- Weight loss: Losing weight, based on a safe and gradual process, may decrease pain and improve function as less compression and excessive wear on the affected joint. - Healthy eating: Nutrient-dense diet that includes adequate minerals (calcium, vitamin D, magnesium), decrease sugary and fatty food, and less sodium intake helps to reduce inflammation, joint pain, stiffness, and improve joint health. - Staying active: Low-impact exercises, stretching, strengthening to improve joint health and to reduce muscle weakness and deconditioning, improve form and posture, and compensatory mechanisms. - Quit smoking: Smoking accelerates OA and cartilage breakdown, affects bone density (leading to increased fracture risk), joint healing after trauma or surgery, doubles heart disease issues, and coronary disease. Proactive measures include addressing muscle weakness due to inactivity, weakness, atrophy (lack of use). Addressing inflammation causing joint swelling, synovitis, cartilage breakdown, tendon and ligament laxity. When people present with these symptoms and muscle disuse muscle weakness, physical therapy is here to address.

While lifestyle modifications or self-care practices are not going to address the underlying pathology, they can have a great impact on the way your body perceives joint-related symptoms and overall comorbidities such as obesity, heart disease, and diabetes. Obesity and high cholesterol may also increase systemic inflammation and OA progression. Focus on both short-term symptom relief as well as long-term benefits of protecting joints by reducing repetitive overloading during activities.

3.4. 4. Surgical Interventions

Surgery plays an important part in the management of neuromuscular diseases. Surgical treatment can restore function, reduce deformity, and assist with physical access and hygiene. The goals of surgery are to improve gait function or ambulation or seating in a wheelchair, to reduce pain, to improve cosmesis, which is the physical appearance of the body, and to address problems of skin breakdown. Procedures often applied to allow functional benefits of the hips and knees for children with cerebral palsy and other neuromuscular conditions should be applied to adults or more chronic conditions. These include maximizing muscle function and addressing problems of deformity or pain.

Surgery is usually considered a last resort, especially for chronic arthritic conditions. Although complications are generally rare, surgery can be costly and time-consuming. Considerations should therefore be made to weigh the benefits and risks of the procedure. Benefits may include the lessening or complete removal of weakness and pain in the joint being operated on. Surgeries can also help patients with weak muscles and, therefore, deformed joints. Unfortunately, surgery does not change the nerve pain caused by the muscle's inability to relax. These painful conditions are often not related to how weak the muscle is, but rather how spastic the muscle is.

Surgical Interventions

4. Preventive Measures and Lifestyle Recommendations

A lifestyle that is supported by a balanced diet and getting healthier can also improve our health and help us prevent weakness, pain, and premature aging. Rest and sleep are also important for supporting recovery and restoring muscle strength. Sufficient rest also affects mental health, leading to a better physiological condition. Such stressless conditions also help reduce the perception or feeling of discomfort. Ease in physical activity will show a good commitment from the client to engage in a variety of physical activities. Often not doing physical activity can also cause sudden weakness. The durability of an individual also changes due to hormonal factors, age, gender, and certain chronic diseases or arthritis. In conclusion, individuals need to be introspective and proactive in maintaining health through various suitable efforts. Holistic aromatherapy massage and reflexology can also be effective in holistic care for arthritis sufferers.

- Engage in proper nutrition, consuming a combination of antioxidants, vitamins, and collagen in a balanced manner. - Keep the body in motion to maintain joint health and reduce the risk of diseases such as arthritis, chronic joint pain, and stiffness. - Maintain a healthy weight by increasing muscle mass, resulting in better bone adaptation to movement and preventing injury. - Keep pain-free through control of chronic joint lupus or weight increase. - Ensure sufficient rest for the recovery of the body as a whole. - Do not work too hard; take a break if feeling tired. Always pay attention to the body's muscle mass, as excessive physical activity can cause tears through the ligaments. Therefore, warm up and cool down after physical activity so that the muscles become more relaxed, reduce tension, and prevent the risk of injury or weakness due to overwork. This can be prevented with a good warm-up and cool-down before and after work. - Use proper protective equipment when playing a supporting role to prevent injury. - Take safety precautions in case of sudden falls, for example, when going upstairs, hold the handlebar, or when walking, support yourself on the road. Always check with your doctor for the best possible treatment that can be given.

Preventive measures & lifestyle recommendations:

5. Conclusion

In conclusion, this paper has shown that patients with joint pain will mostly suffer from weakness in one or several muscles surrounding the painful joint. Furthermore, the risk of suffering from pain in a joint increases with the presence of muscle weakness, and vice versa, the risk of weakness in a muscle increases with the presence of pain in that muscle. However, these possible relationships cannot be recommended as a policy of treating patients with one of the two conditions as a preventer of the other. Future RCTs are needed to clarify the issue of the effect of joint pain treatment and tylosis on muscle weakness and vice versa.

In this essay, we discussed seven different potential relationships that joint pain and weakness have and presented evidence and opinions about these options. However, apart from the quadriceps weakness caused by pain in PFJ, and vice versa (quadriceps weakness causing PFJ pain), very little good-quality evidence exists for the relationships between joint pain and muscle weakness. The principal area of interest appears to be weakness that develops from the onset of joint pain, although cause and effect is incredibly hard to demonstrate. We have also discussed treatment strategies based on some evidence and expert opinion for the conditions described in this essay.

Joint pain and weakness are extremely common and have an important relationship. Joint pain not only reduces function and quality of life but changes the alignment and loading of joints, thus leading to weakness. Conversely, weakness increases the risk of joint injury and subsequently pain.